FINGER ACU*PRESSURE*

"During my recent trip to China, I witnessed treatment using finger pressure for relieving toothache or tooth extraction. The method is simple, easy, and causes no pain to the patient . . . There is definitely some relation and connection between point(s) of skin and disorder(s) of the human body. The question is to get them stimulated. There are quite a number of ways of stimulation, such as needles, moxa, electricity, injection or even *finger pressure*."

—James Y. P. Chen, M.D.

Pedro Chan is an Acupuncture Research Associate at White Memorial Medical Center in Los Angeles and the author of *Wonders of Chinese Acupuncture*.

FINGER ACUPRESSURE*

Treatment for Many Common Ailments
from Insomnia to Impotence
By Using Finger Massage on Acupuncture Points

PEDRO CHAN

*Finger Acupuncture

Formerly published as *Finger Acupressure: Treatment for
Many Common Ailments From Migraine to Insomnia
By Using Finger Massage on Acupuncture Points*

BALLANTINE BOOKS • NEW YORK

Library of Congress Catalog Card Number: 74-76761

ISBN 0-345-30285-0

This edition published by arrangement with Price/Stern/Sloane Publishers, Inc.

Manufactured in the United States of America

First Ballantine Books Edition: February 1975
Seventh Printing: June 1981

CONTENTS

FOREWORD

Acupuncture is an ancient Chinese art of healing by inserting fine needles in the body at certain well-defined points. The idea that a fine needle pricking the skin at the back of the knee (Wei-chung, Bladder 54) can in a few minutes relieve a long-standing low-back pain; that one painlessly piercing a point on the back of the hand near the base of the thumb (Ho-ku, Large intestine 4) can relieve toothache or even induce anesthesia for tonsillectomy; or that one placed in the skin about three inches below the kneecap just outside the tibia (Tsu-san-li, Stomach 36) can relieve stomach ache, cure gastritis, combat general fatigue and, at the same time, conserve robust health, may sound fantastic to the Western mind. Nonetheless, the experience of those knowledgeable in acupuncture either as a doctor, patient, or objective observer seems to confirm some, at least, of these claims.

There are some 500 to 800 acupuncture points or spots as shown by various Chinese and Japanese charts. Exactly 669 points are listed in Dr. Chu Lien's *Hsin Chen Chiu Hsueh* (*Modern Acupuncture*), a standard textbook on acupuncture used in present-day China. Many new points have been discovered in China in recent years. There is definitely some relation and connection between point(s) of skin and disorder(s) of the human body. The question is to get them stimulated. There are quite a number of ways of stimulation, such as needles, moxa, electricity, injection—and finger pressure.

During my recent trip to China, I witnessed treatments using finger pressure for relieving toothache or tooth extraction. The method is simple, easy, and causes no pain to the patient. Mr. Pedro Chan, an associate of mine in Chinese medicine, has used his experience, and others', to illustrate with simplicity the essence of finger acupuncture (acupressure). This appears to be the first guidebook of such a technique in the English language, and should be a good guide for those beginners without previous knowledge of acupuncture.

James Y. P. Chen, M.D.
Vice President, American Society
    of Chinese Medicine
President, Acupuncture Research Institute

INTRODUCTION

The word *acupuncture* comes from two Latin words: *acus* and *punctura*. Acus means needle; puncture means pricking. The term describes the Chinese art of healing involving the insertion of needles into specific points of the body, called acupuncture points. Finger acupressure, as the name implies, is a kind of healing which involves finger massage over the acupuncture points.

The origin of acupuncture and acupressure is shrouded in antiquity. According to tradition, some 5,000 years ago the Chinese noticed that pain could be relieved when they rubbed stones against their bodies. They also discovered that some soldiers, having been wounded by arrows, recovered from long-suffered illness. This collection of ideas led to the principle that stimulation of various points of the body, either by pressure or by insertion of needles, could benefit sufferers of many diseases and common ailments. This can be said to be the beginning of acupuncture and acupressure.

The author, using his own experience as well as that of other professionals, has picked out those acupuncture points most effective for treating certain common disorders using the finger technique. It is simple, easy, harmless, and effective in most cases. It can be used anywhere and by anyone without special knowledge. Subjects will not be scared because there is no needle insertion. From a practical standpoint this treatment can be applied as a first-aid measure because of its efficacy and convenience. Also, no equipment or drug is needed in the procedure.

However, finger acupressure is never a cure. It is also not the intention of the author to provide a sub-

stitute for acupuncture or conventional therapy. Finger acupressure should only be used as a supplement. By all means, see a licensed acupuncturist or physician for any condition requiring medical treatment.

PEDRO CHAN
Los Angeles, California
1974

THE ESSENTIALS OF FINGER ACUPRESSURE

Posture

No matter what the subject's posture is—lying down or sitting up—he or she must be relaxed, comfortable, and natural. The practitioner must be able to utilize fully his finger movement and strength.

Finger Pressure

The degree of pressure varies with the condition and physique of the subject. Generally, light pressure is applied on subjects in the following categories:

1. First-time subject
2. When there is acute pain
3. Where there is swelling
4. When the muscles are weak or loose
5. When there are complications such as high blood pressure, severe anemia, or heart trouble.

Hard pressure is applied on subjects who:

1. Have a chronic problem
2. Have no other complications
3. Are not overly tired

Manipulation

Press against the designated point on the skin surface. Massage in a small circular movement, about two or three cycles per second. It is preferable to apply pressure bilaterally. Start with one point at a time, and when you master this technique, you may work bilaterally and simultaneously with your two hands.

Period of Treatment

This can range from one minute to five minutes for each point per treatment. Treatment can be once a day, whenever you have the problem, or whenever you wish to do it.

Caution

Please keep the following in mind:

1. Keep the treatment room warm but well ventilated. This will help the subject to be comfortable and prevent him or her from becoming chilled.
2. The practitioner should keep his hands clean and warm and his nails trimmed to prevent injuring the subject or making him or her nervous and tense.
3. Never work on a subject who has a full stomach.
4. The treatment is not to be applied on pregnant women or serious cardiac patients.
5. Avoid working on skin surface where there is contusion, scar, or infection.
6. Stop treatment if the symptom is being aggravated and no relief is observed.

Forbidden Diet

Diet plays an important role in Chinese medicine,

as some foods have certain counter or irritating effects on the patient. It is wise, therefore, to avoid the following foods during treatment:

1. Iced food or drink
2. Sour foods, such as vinegar, pickle, lemon, or pineapple
3. Alcoholic drinks
4. Irritating foods, such as pepper, hot sauce, or spices
5. Seafood with shells, such as lobster, shrimp, or crab

ALPHABETICAL LIST OF DISORDERS

Simplicity is the main feature of this book.

Listed under each disorder is the name of the acupuncture point (with its meridian) where pressure is to be applied and a description of its location. This is further illustrated by:

1. A drawing of the anatomical location, with relation to skeletal structure;
2. A picture showing live treatment.

Follow the instruction and diagram to locate the correct point. Press firmly and deeply. If this is done correctly, the subject should feel some numbness, soreness, swelling, and heaviness.

Note: For some ailments, it is necessary to use pressure on more than one acupuncture point. In this case, when more than one point is shown, use them one by one.

Point

Tsu-san-li
(Bladder 36)

Location

About 3 inches below the knee-cap, 1 inch lateral to the tibia.

Technique

Subject should lie or sit down. Use thumb to press down, then massage upward.

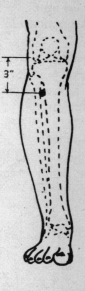

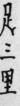

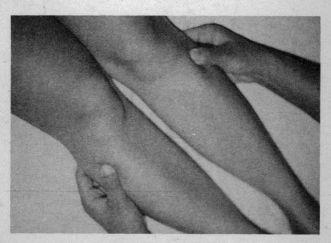

Point
Chung-wan
(Conception 12)

Location
About 4 inches above the navel, along the midline of the abdominal surface.

Technique
Subject should lie or sit down. Use thumb or palm to massage inward.

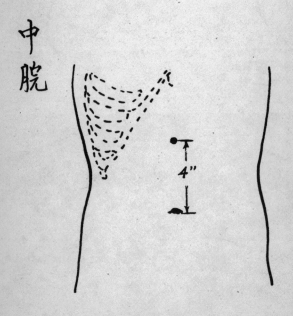

中脘

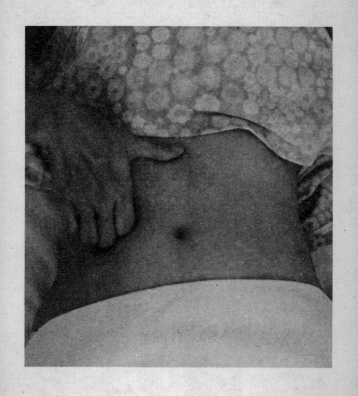

Point

Ho-ku
(Large Intestine 4)

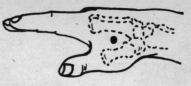

Location

Over the dorsum of the hand, in between the 1st and 2nd metacarpal bones.

Technique

Subject should lie or sit down. Use thumb to press against the 2nd metacarpal bone.

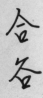

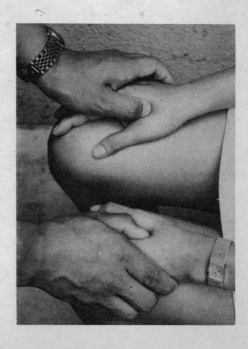

Point
Kun-lun
(Bladder 60)

Location
In the depression behind the lateral ankle.

Technique
Subject should lie or sit down.
Use thumb to press hard.

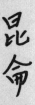

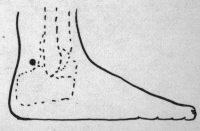

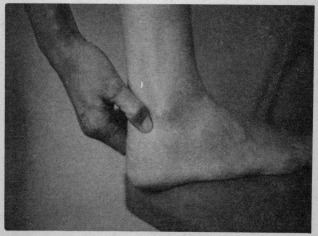

Point

Tien-tu

(Conception 22)

Location

In the depression above the su-
prasternal notch.

Technique

Subject should lie or sit down.
Use index finger to press inward,
then massage downward.

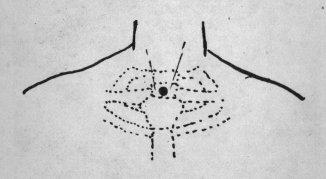

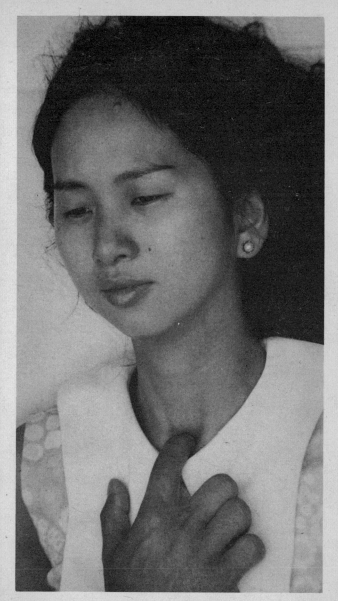

Point
Chuan-hsi
(New Point)

Location
About 1 inch lateral to the lower
end of the 7th cervical disk.

Technique
Subject should sit down and bend
the head forward.
Use thumb to massage hard toward the disk.

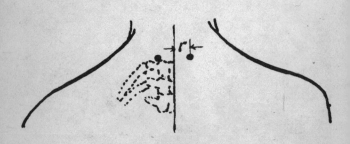

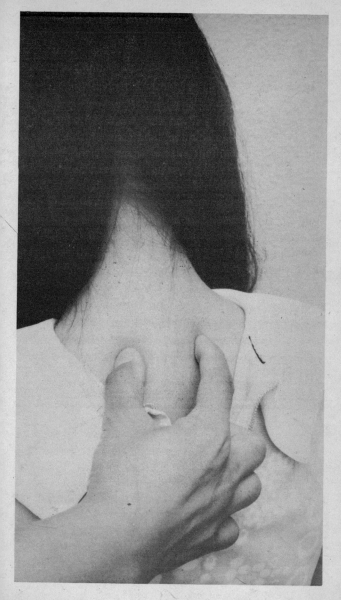

Point
Fei-shu
(Bladder 13)

Location
About 1.5 inches lateral to the lower end of the 3rd thoracic disk.

Technique
Subject should sit down or lie down on the stomach.
Use thumb to massage hard toward the disk.

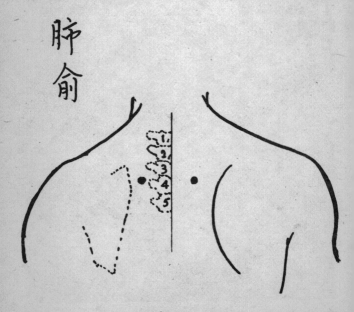

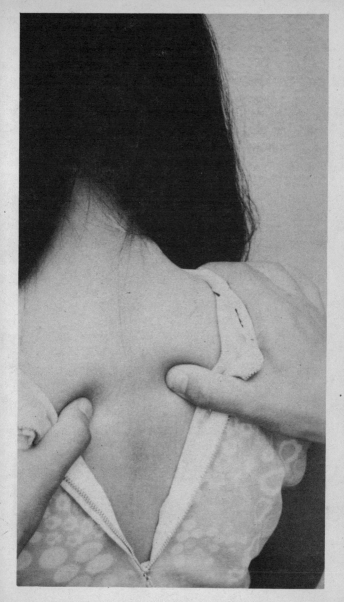

Point

Kao-huang
(Bladder 38)

Location

About 3 inches lateral to the lower end of the 4th thoracic disk.

Technique

Subject should sit down or lie down on the stomach.
Use thumb to massage hard.

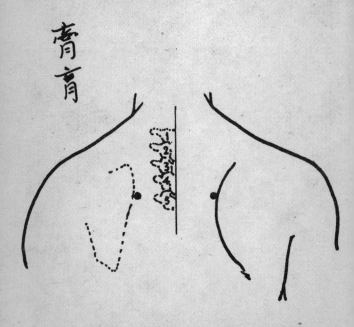

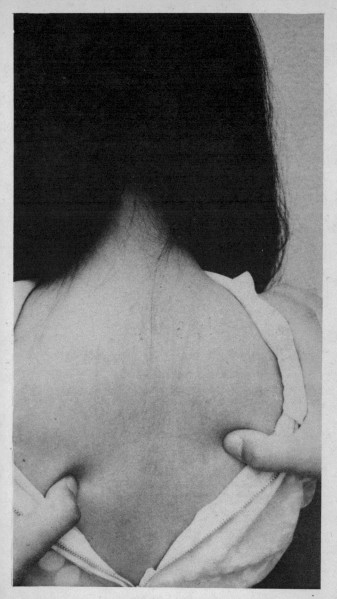

Point
Nocturia
(New Point)

Location
In the centers of the little finger creases.

Technique
Subject should lie or sit down. Use thumbnail to press hard. Try point #1 first; if no result, try points #1 and #2.

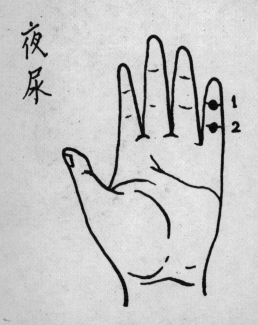

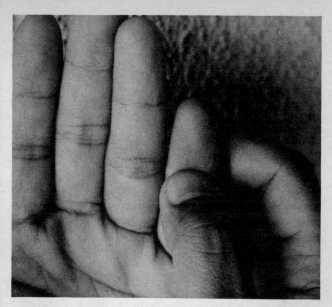

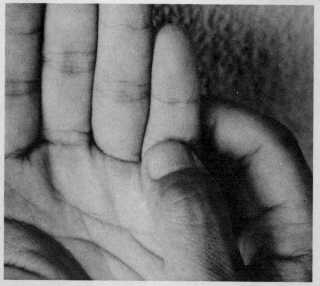

Point
Ear lobe
(New point)

Location
In the center of the ear lobe.

Technique
Subject can assume any posture. Take the ear lobe between the thumb and index finger and press.

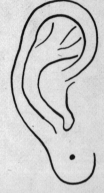

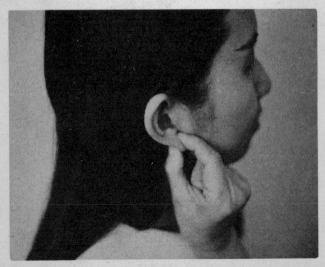

Point
Ho-ku
(Large Intestine 4)

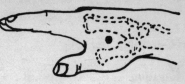

Location
Over the dorsum of the hand, in between the 1st and 2nd meta-carpal bones.

Technique
Subject should lie or sit down.
Use thumb to press against the 2nd metacarpal bone.

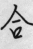

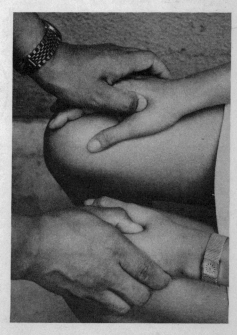

Point
Ta-chui
(Governing 14)

Location
In between the 7th cervical and the 1st thoracic vertebrae.

Technique
Subject should sit or lie down on his side. The head should be bent down slightly.
Use the tip of the index finger to press and massage.

大椎

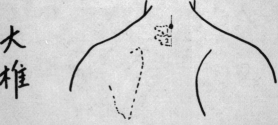

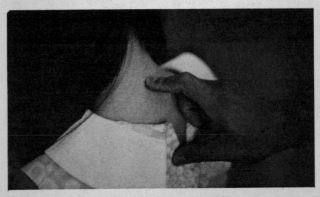

Common cold (*continued*)

Point
Feng-men
(Bladder 12)

Location
About 1.5 inches lateral to the lower end of the 2nd thoracic vertebra.

Technique
Subject should sit or lie down on his side.
Use thumb to massage.

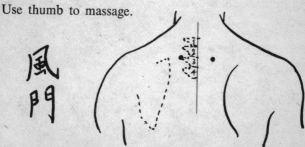

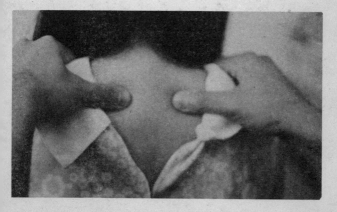

Point
Tien-tu
(Conception 22)

Location
In the depression above the su-
prasternal notch.

Technique
Subject should sit or lie down.
Use index finger to press inward,
then massage downward.

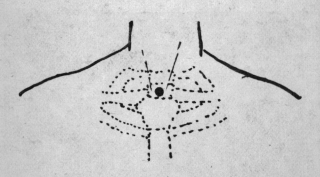

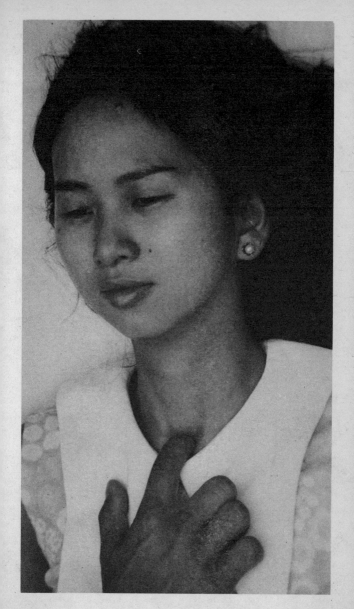

Point

Chu-chih
(Large Intestine 11)

Location

At the external end of the elbow
crease when it's bent at 90°.

Technique

Subject should sit or lie down.
Use thumb to press hard.

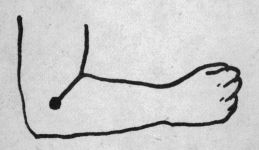

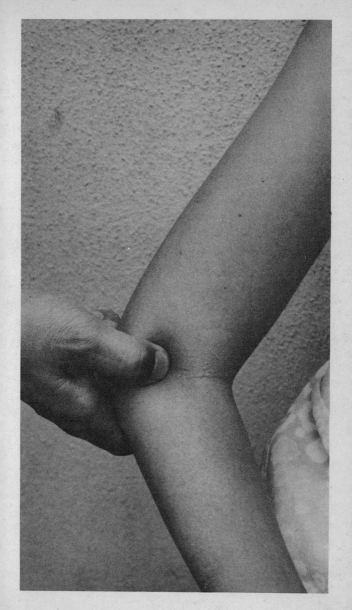

Point
Chung-chi

Location
About 4 inches below the navel, along the midline of the abdominal surface.

Technique
Subject should lie down.
Use thumb or palm to press hard.

中
極

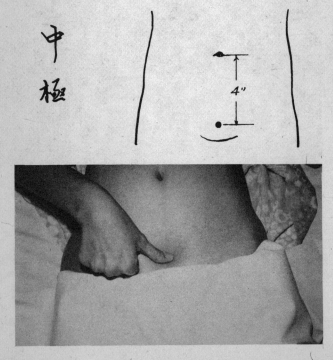

Point
Chang-chiang

Location
In between the tip of the tail-bone and the anus.

Technique
Subject should lie down on stomach.
Use index finger to press downward, then massage upward.

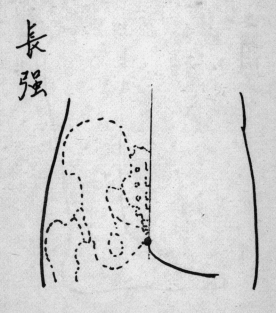

Point

San-yin-chiao
(Spleen 6)

Location

About 3 inches above the medial
ankle, behind the tibia.

Technique

Subject should sit or lie down.
Use thumb to press hard.

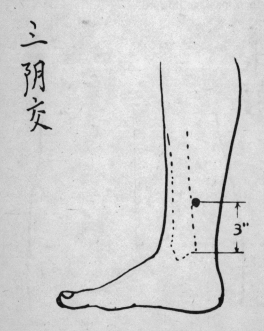

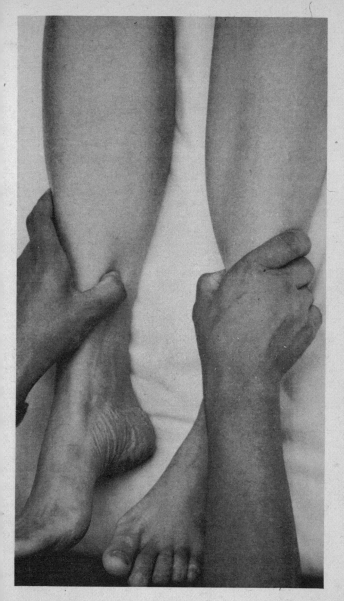

Point
Chih-yin
(Bladder 67)

Location
About 1/10 of an inch behind
the lateral corner of the little toe
nail.

Technique
Subject should lie down.
Use thumbnail to press down.

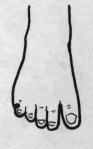

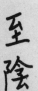

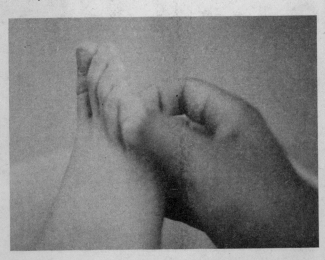

Dizziness

Point
Yin-tang
(Non-meridian point)

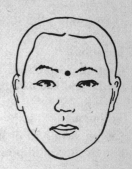

Location
In between the eyebrows.

Technique
Subject should sit or lie down.
Use thumb and index finger to
pinch hard.

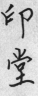

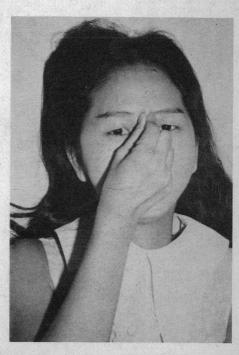

Point
Tai-chung
(Liver 3)

Location
Over the depression in between the 1st and 2nd metatarsal bones.

Technique
Subject should sit or lie down. Use thumbnail to press hard.

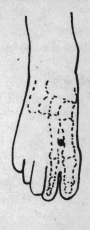

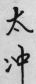

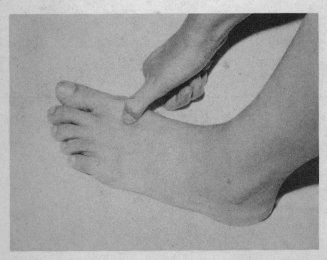

Point

Tongue-tip *

Location

At the tip of the tongue.

Technique

Subject can assume any posture. Use front teeth to bite the tip of the tongue, and swallow the saliva. (This is obviously done by the subject on himself.)

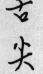

---

* This is not an acupuncture point.

Point
Chu-chih
(Large Intestine 11)

Location
At the external end of the elbow
crease when the elbow is bent at
90°.

Technique
Subject should sit or lie down.
Use thumb to press hard.

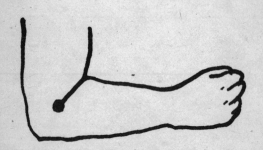

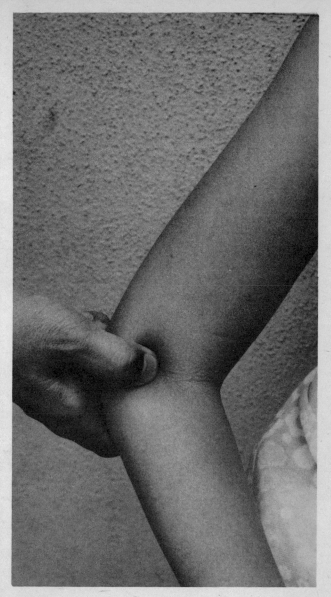

Point
Jan-chung
(Governing 26)

Location
Just above the middle of philtrum.

Technique
Subject should sit or lie down.
Use thumbnail or index fingernail to press hard.

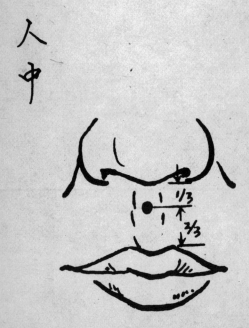

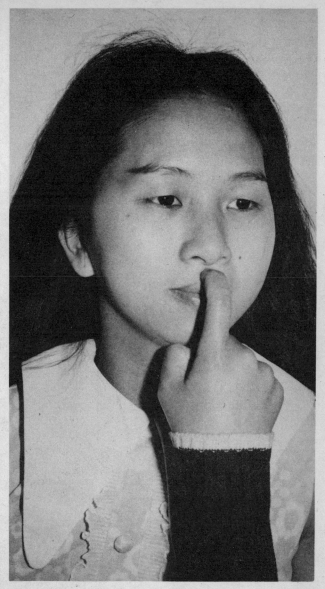

Point

Yung-chuan
(Kidney 1)

Location

At the anterior third of the sole, between the 2nd and 3rd metatarsal bones.

Technique

Subject should lie down.
Use thumbnail to press hard.

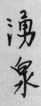

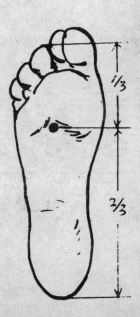

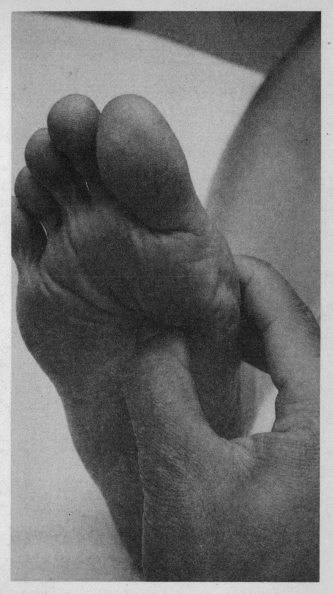

Point

Ho-ku
(Large Intestine 4)

Location
Over the dorsum of the hand, in between the 1st and 2nd metacarpal bones.

Technique
Subject should sit or lie down. Use thumb to press against the 2nd metacarpal bone.

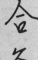
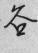

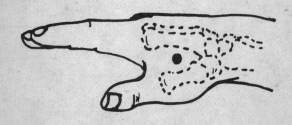

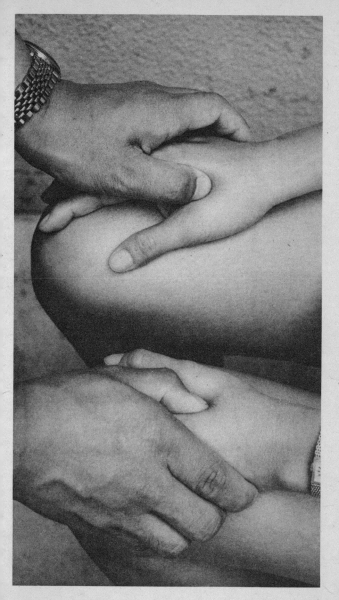

Point
Feng-chih
(Gall Bladder 20)

Location
Below the occipital bone, about
1.5 inches lateral to the midline
of the head.

Technique
Subject should sit down and bend
the head forward.
Use thumb to massage hard.

風
池

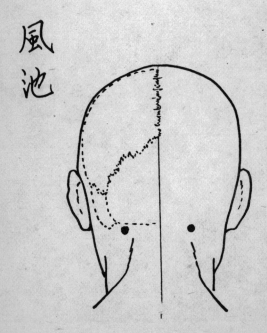

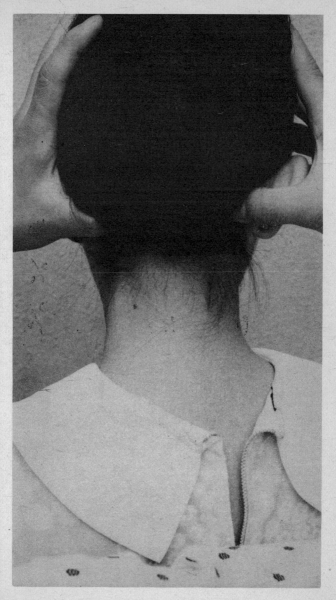

Point
Jan-chung
(Governing 26)

Location
Just above the middle of philtrum.

Technique
Subject should sit or lie down.
Use thumbnail or index finger-
nail to press hard.

人
中

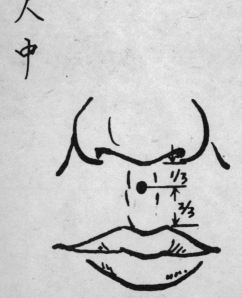

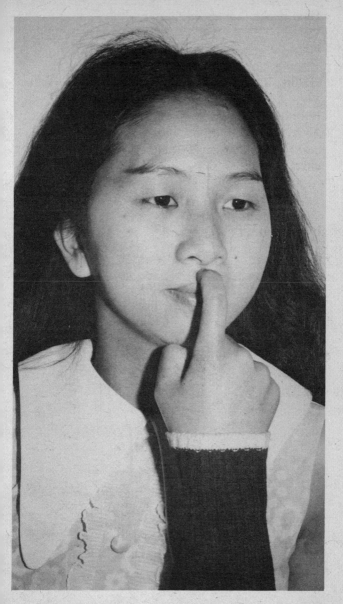

59

Point

Yung-chuan
(Kidney 1)

Location

At the anterior third of the sole,
between the 2nd and 3rd metatarsal bones.

Technique

Subject should lie down.
Use thumbnail to press hard.

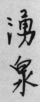

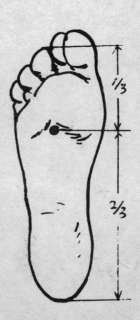

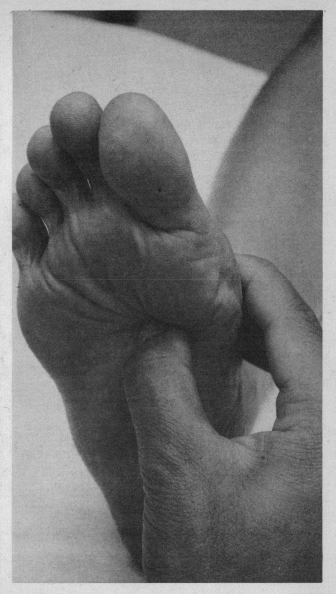

61

Point
Vertex
(New point)

Location
On the radial side of the dorsal surface of the phalangeal joint of the middle finger.

Technique
Subject can assume any posture. Use the thumbnail to press hard.

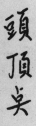

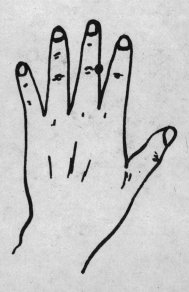

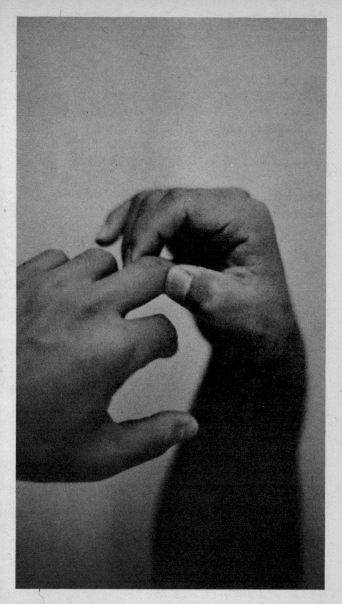

Point
Ke-shu
(Bladder 17)

Location
About 1.5 inches lateral to the lower end of the 7th thoracic vertebra.

Technique
Subject should sit or lie down on side.
Use thumb to press down hard.

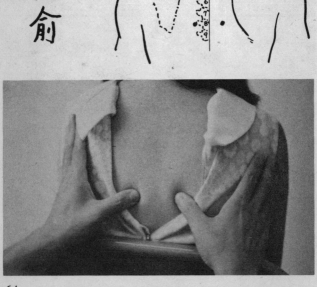

Hypertension

Point
Jen-ying
(Stomach 9)

Location
About 1.5 inches lateral to the Adam's Apple.

Technique
Subject should sit or lie down. Use thumb and index finger to press both points at the same time. Do not exert excess force.

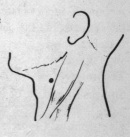

人迎

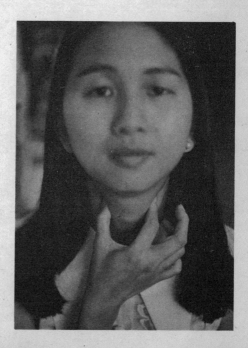

Point
Blood pressure point
(New point)

Location
About 2 inches lateral to the lower end of the 6th cervical vertebra.

Technique
Subject should sit or lie down on side.
Use thumbs to press and massage both points.

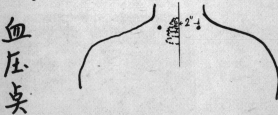

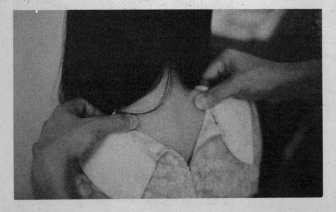

Point

Depressing Groove
(New point)

Location

A curved vertical groove on the
back of the ear.

Technique

Subject can assume any posture.
Use fingernail to press down
hard.

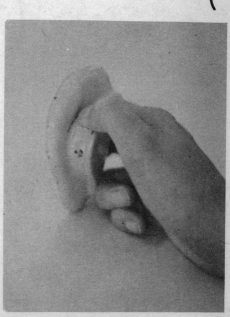

降
压
沟

Point
Hysteria
(New point)

Location
At the center of the bottom
crease of the thumb.

Technique
Subject can assume any posture.
Use thumbnail to press hard.

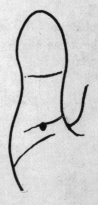

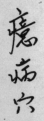

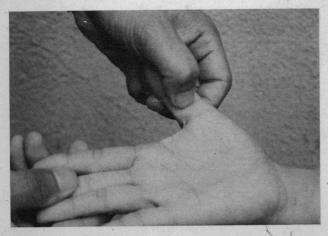

Point
*Penis**

Location
At the tip of the penis.

Technique
Subject can assume any comfortable posture.
Use thumb and index finger to squeeze the tip of the penis, while the penis is still erect before orgasm.

* This is not an acupuncture point. Needle insertion is prohibited.

Point
Kuan-yuan
(Conception 4)

Location
About 3 inches below the navel,
along the midline of the abdominal surface.

Technique
Subject should lie down.
Use thumb or palm to massage
hard.

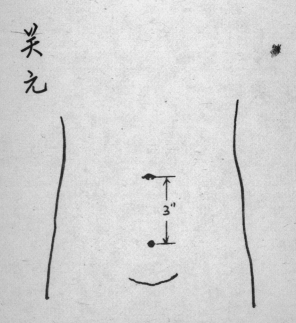

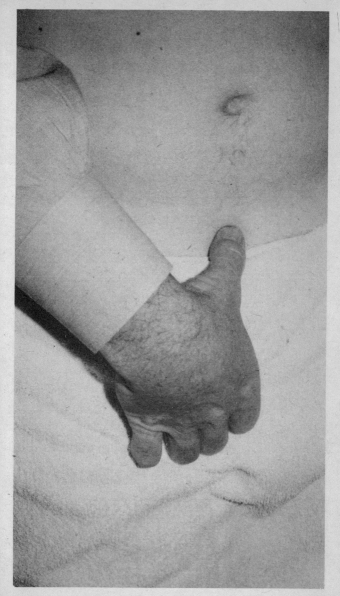

Point

San-yin-chiao
(Spleen 6)

Location

About 3 inches above the medial
ankle, behind the tibia.

Technique

Subject should lie down.
Use thumb to press hard.

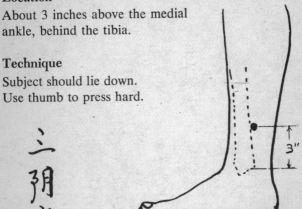

三
陰
交

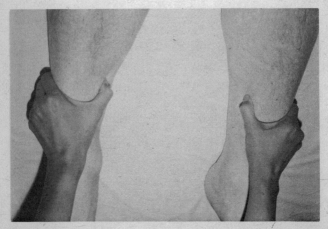

Point

Tsu-san-li
(Stomach 36)

Location

About 3 inches below the knee-cap, 1 inch lateral to the tibia.

Technique

Subject should lie down.
Use thumb to press down, then massage upward.

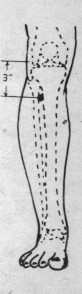

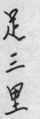

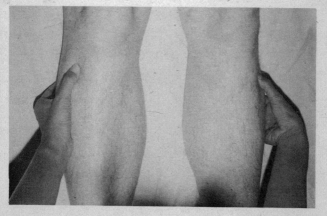

Point
Shen-shu
(Bladder 23)

Location
About 1.5 inches lateral to the lower end of the 2nd lumbar disk.

Technique
Subject should lie down on stomach.
Use thumb to press hard toward spine.

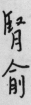

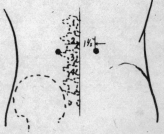

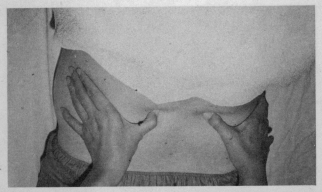

Insomnia

Point
An-mien
(New point)

Location
About 1 inch behind the lobule
of the ear.

Technique
Subject should sit or lie down.
Use index finger to press hard.
(If this point does not work, see
next page.)

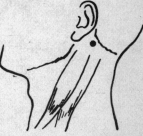

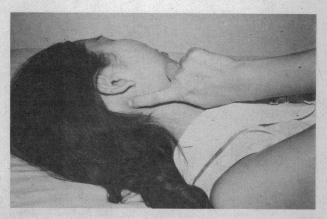

Point
Shen-man
(Heart 7)

Location
Along the most distal skin crease
of the wrist, on the ulnar side,
medial to the tendon.

Technique
Subject should sit or lie down.
Use thumbnail to press hard.

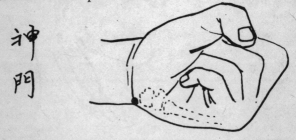

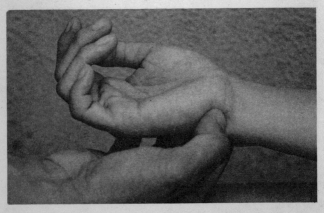

Point

San-yin-chiao
(Spleen 6)

Location

About 3 inches above the medial
ankle, behind the tibia.

Technique

Subject should sit or lie down.
Use thumb to press hard.

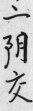

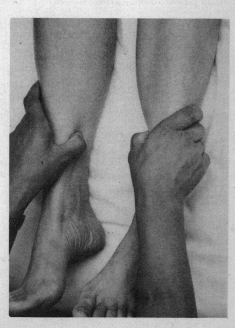

Knee pain

Point
Chi-yen
(Stomach 35)

Location
In the two depressions below the kneecap.

Technique
Subject should sit down and bend the knee.
Use thumb and index finger to press hard at the two depressions at the same time.

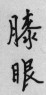

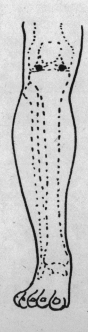

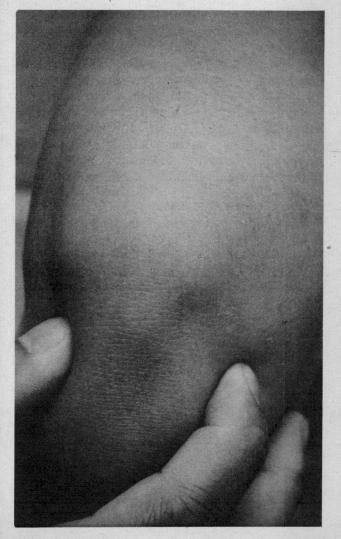

Point
Yang-ling-chuan
(Gall bladder 34)

Location
About 2 inches below the knee-
cap, just in front of the fibula.

Technique
Subject should sit down and bend
the knee.
Use thumb to press hard.

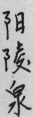

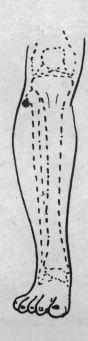

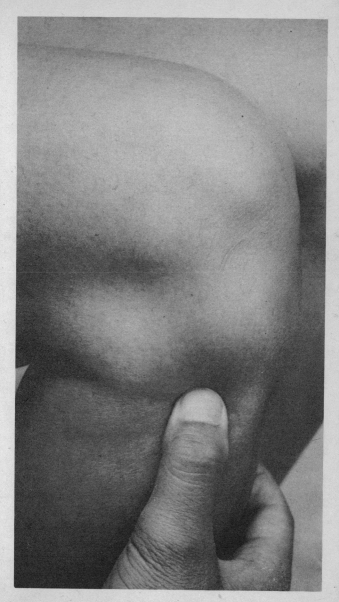

Point
Chia-che
(Stomach 6)

Location
Over the masseteric muscle.

Technique
Subject should sit or lie down. Use both thumbs to massage both points at the same time.

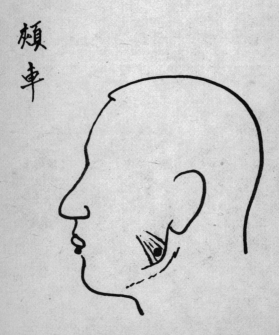

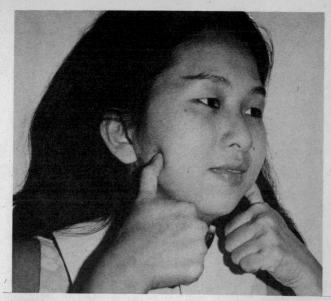

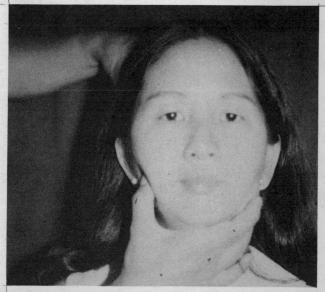

Point
Shen-shu
(Bladder 23)

Location
About 1.5 inches lateral to the lower end of the 2nd lumbar disk.

Technique
Subject should lie down on stomach.
Use thumb to press hard toward the spine.

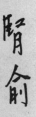

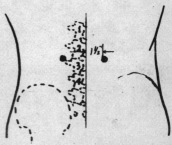

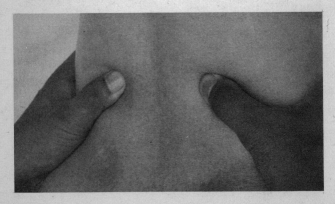

Point
An-mien
(New point)

Location
About 1 inch behind the lobule
of the ear.

Technique
Subject should sit or lie down.
Use index finger to press hard.

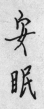

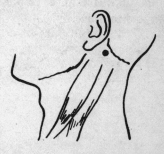

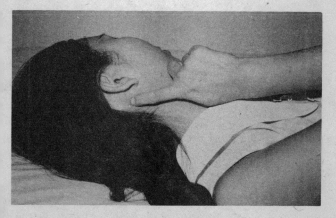

Point
Nei-kuan
(Pericardium 6)

Location
About 2 inches above the middle of the palmar wrist crease, in between the two tendons.

Technique
Subject may assume any posture. Use the tip of the finger to press down and massage.

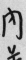

内
关

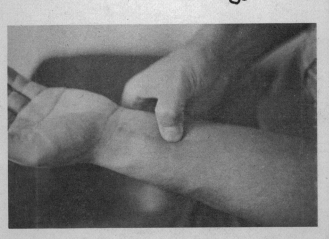

Point

Tsu-san-li
(Stomach 36)

Location

About 3 inches below the knee-cap, 1 inch lateral to the tibia.

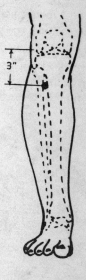

Technique

Subject should lie down.
Use thumb to press down, then massage upward.

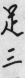

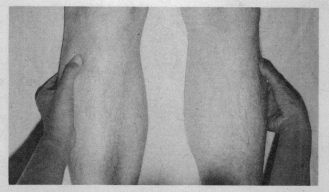

Point

San-yin-chiao
(Spleen 6)

Location

About 3 inches above the medial
ankle, behind the tibia.

Technique

Subject should sit or lie down.
Use thumb to press hard.

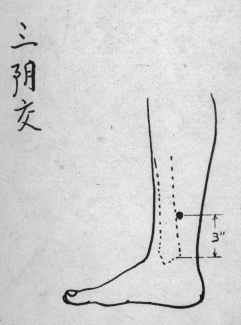

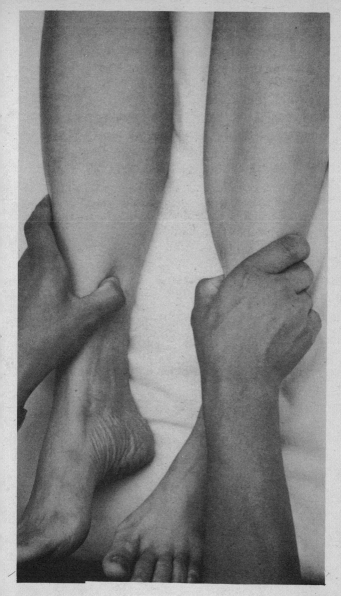

Point

Shen-man
(Heart 7)

Location

Along the most distal crease of
the wrist, on the ulnar side, medial to the tendon.

Technique

Subject should sit or lie down.
Use thumbnail to press hard.

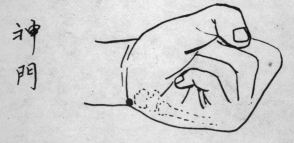

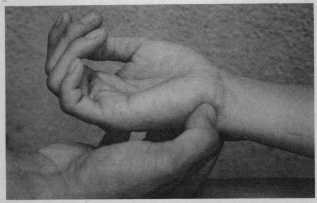

Palpitation

Point
Shen-man
(Heart 7)

Location
Along the most distal crease of the wrist, on the ulnar side, medial to the tendon.

Technique
Subject should sit or lie down. Use thumbnail to press hard.

神
門

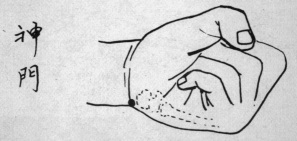

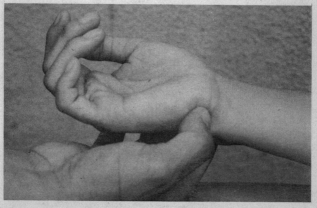

Point

Tien-tu

(Conception 22)

Location

In the depression above the su-
prasternal notch.

Technique

Subject should sit or lie down.
Use index finger to press inward,
then massage downward.

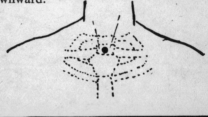

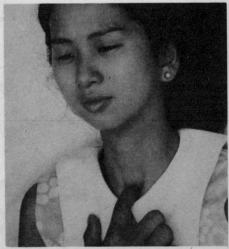

Point
Chuan-hsi
(New point)

Location
About 1 inch lateral to the lower
end of the 7th cervical disk.

Technique
Subject should sit down and bend
the head forward.
Use thumb to massage hard toward the disk.

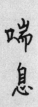

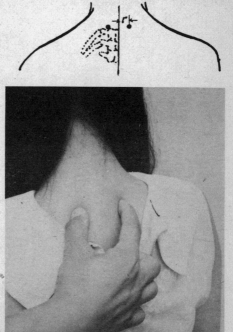

Point
Fei-shu
(Bladder 13)

Location
About 1.5 inches lateral to the lower end of the 3rd thoracic disk.

Technique
Subject should sit down or lie down on stomach.
Use thumb to massage hard toward the disk.

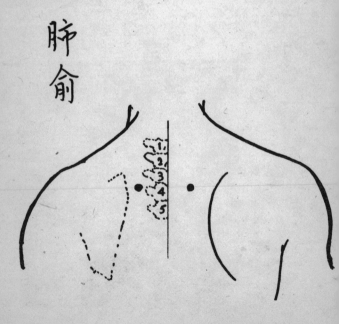

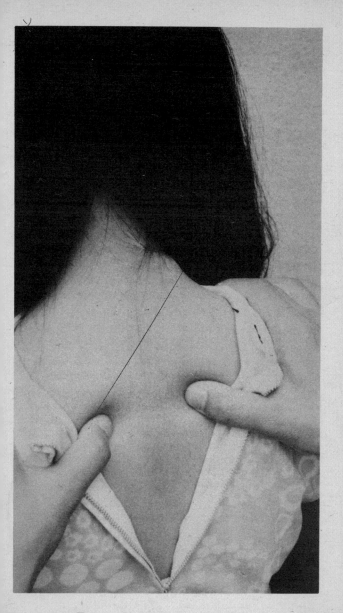

Point
Kao-huáng
(Bladder 38)

Location
About 3 inches lateral to the lower end of the 4th thoracic disk.

Technique
Subject should sit down or lie down on stomach.
Use thumb to massage hard.

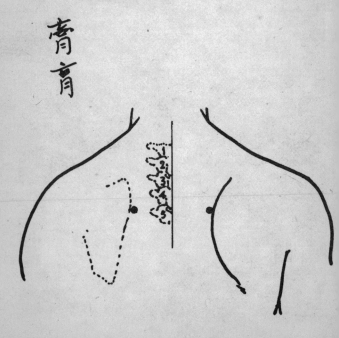

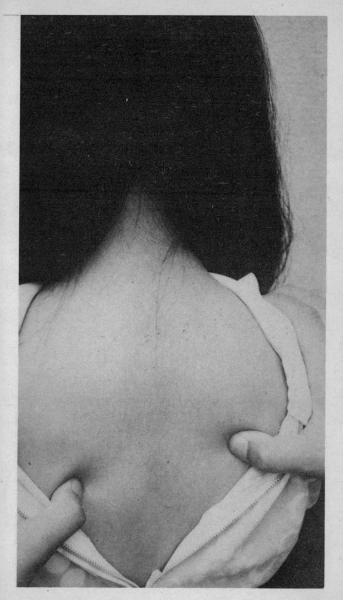

Pedotic (children's) pot belly

Point
Szu-feng
(Non-meridian point)

Location
On the palmar surface, the middle of the proximal joint crease of each of the four fingers.

Technique
Subject may assume any posture. Use the fingernail to press down.

四縫

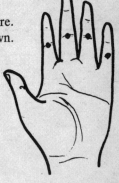

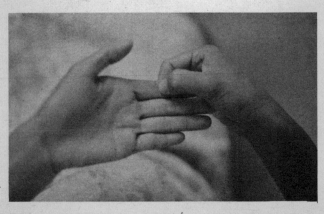

Shoulder pain

Point
Chien-yu
(Large Intestine 15)

Location
At the antero-inferior part of the shoulder.

Technique
Subject should sit down.
Use thumb to press hard.

肩
髃

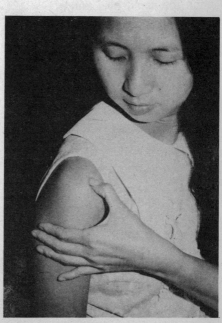

Point
Chien-chin
(Gall Bladder 21)

Location
On the hump of the shoulder, along the same vertical line with the nipple.

Technique
Subject should sit down.
Use thumb over Chien-chin and the other fingers over shoulder to squeeze and release. Repeat this action for about one minute.

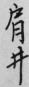

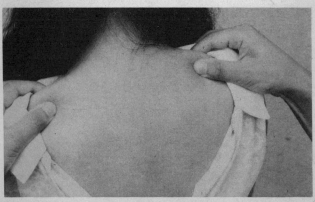

Sinus pain

Point
Yin-tang
(Non-meridian point)

Location
In between the eyebrows.

Technique
Subject should sit or lie down.
Use thumb and index finger to
pinch hard.

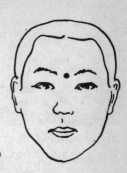

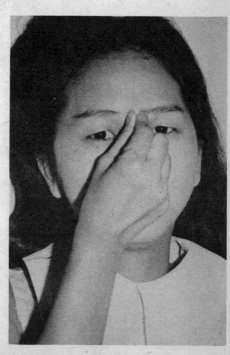

Point

Ying-hsiang
(Large Intestine 20)

Location

By the side of the nose.

Technique

Subject should sit or lie down.
Use index finger to massage.

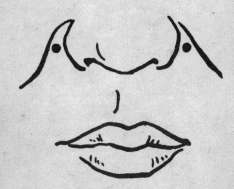

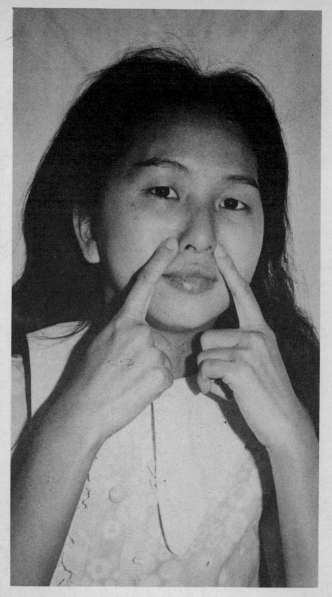

Point
Shao-shang
(Lung 11)

Location
About 0.1 inch away from the corner of the thumbnail.

Technique
Subject may assume any posture. Use thumbnail to press hard.

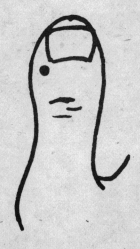

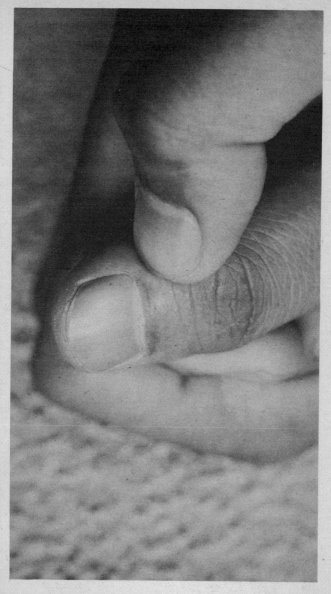

Point
Ho-ku
(Large Intestine 4)

Location
Over the dorsum of the hand, in between the 1st and 2nd meta-carpal bone.

Technique
Subject may assume any posture. Use thumb to press hard against the 2nd metacarpal bone.

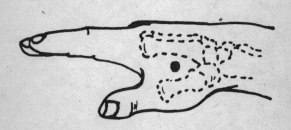

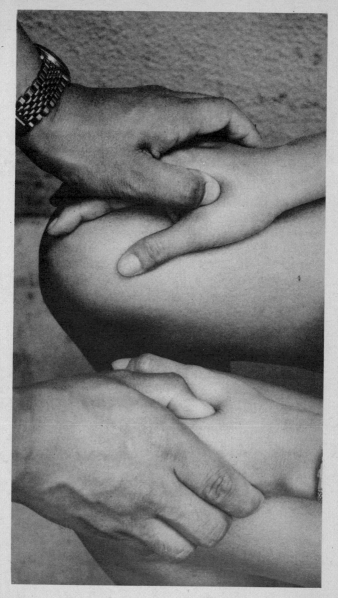

Point

Feng-chih
(Gall Bladder 20)

Location

Below the occipital bone, about
1.5 inches lateral to the midline
of the head.

Technique

Subject should sit down and bend
the head forward.
Use thumb to massage hard.

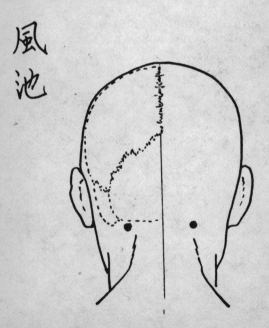

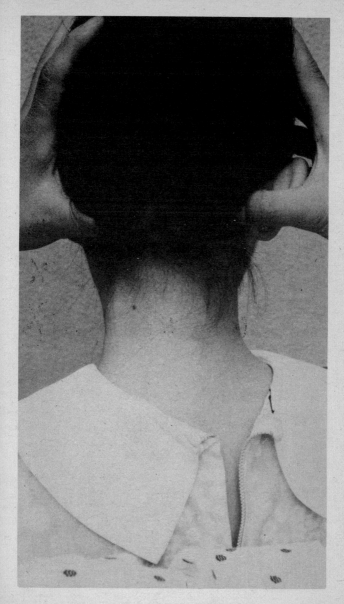

Point
Chien-chin
(Gall Bladder 21)

Location
On the hump of the shoulder,
along the same vertical line with
the nipple.

Technique
Subject should sit down.
Use thumb over Chien-chin and
the other fingers over shoulder
to squeeze and release. Repeat
this action for about one minute.

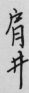

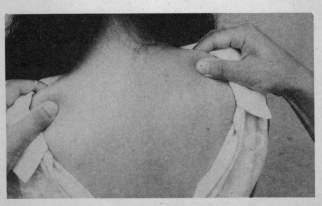

Point
Jan-chung
(Governing 26)

Location
Just above the middle of philtrum.

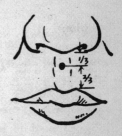

Technique
Subject should sit or lie down.
Use thumbnail or index finger to
press hard.

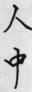

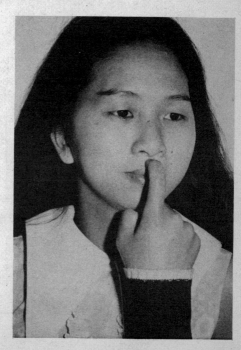

Point

Yung-chuan
(Kidney 1)

Location

At the anterior third of the sole,
between the 2nd and 3rd metatarsal bones.

Technique

Subject should lie down.
Use thumbnail to press hard.

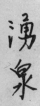

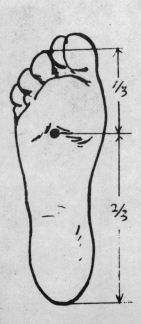

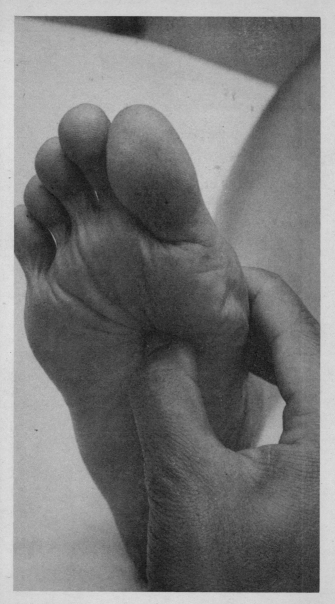

Point
Polyhidrosis
(New point)

Location
At the center of the palm.

Technique
Subject should sit or lie down.
Use thumbnail to press hard.

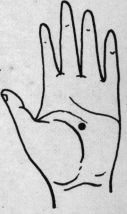

多
汗

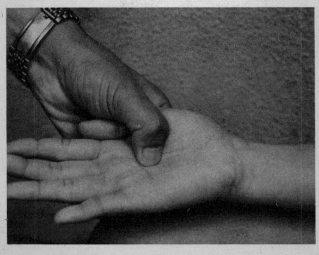

Point
Jan-chung
(Governing 26)

Location
Just above the middle of philtrum.

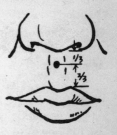

Technique
Subject should sit or lie down.
Use thumbnail or index finger-
nail to press hard.

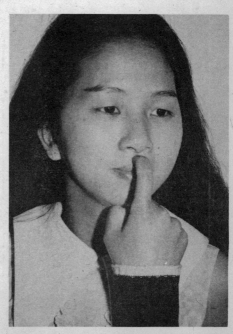

Point

Yung-chuan

(Kidney 1)

Location

At the anterior third of the sole,
between the 2nd and 3rd metatarsal bones.

Technique

Subject should lie down.
Use thumbnail to press hard.

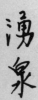

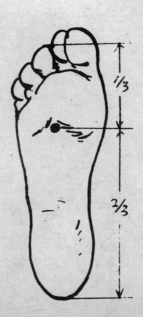

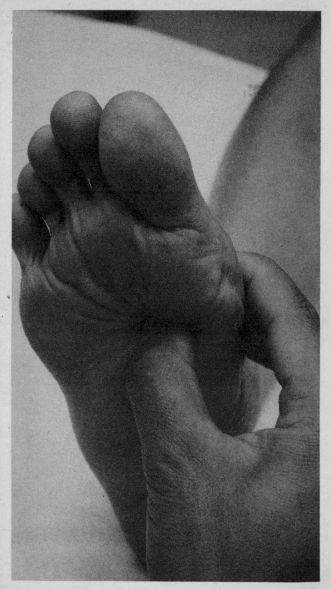

Point

Ho-ku
(Large Intestine 4)

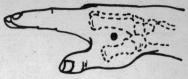

Location

Over the dorsum of the hand, in between the 1st and 2nd meta-carpal bone.

Technique

Subject should sit or lie down. Use thumb to press against the 2nd metacarpal bone.

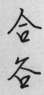

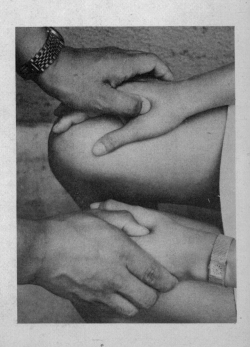

Point

Hsia-kuan
(Stomach 7)

Location

In the depression about 1 inch in front of the tragus.

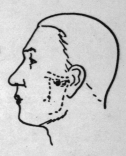

Technique

Subject should sit or lie down. Use thumb to press hard.

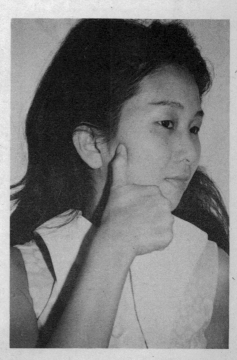

Point
Chia-che
(Stomach 6)

Location
Over the masseteric muscle.

Technique
Subject should sit or lie down.
Use thumb to massage hard.

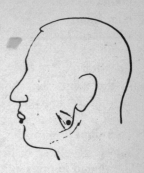

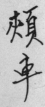

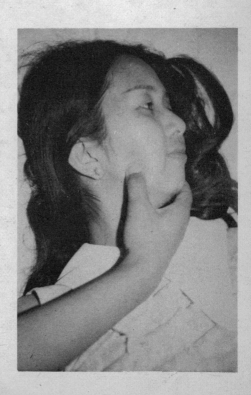

Point

Tongue-tip *

Location

At the tip of the tongue.

Technique

Subject may assume any posture.
Use front teeth to bite the tip of
the tongue, and swallow the saliva.

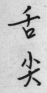

* This is not an acupuncture point.

Point

Yang-lao
(Small Intestine 6)

Location

Along the seam on the radial side
of the distal head of the ulna.

Technique

Subject may assume any posture.
Use fingernail to press down
hard.

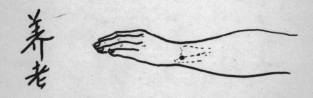

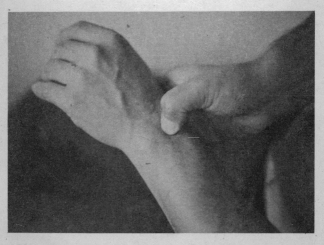

ACUPRESSURE FOR GOOD HEALTH AND PREVENTING DISEASES *

While acupressure can be used to control certain diseases and ailments and to enhance the therapeutic effect of other agents, it can also be employed to help prevent diseases and strengthen the health. The following twenty procedures can be used either individually, according to your situation, or all of them can be used. For preventing diseases and strengthening physical health, do the procedures upon rising in the morning or before sleeping at night. For certain diseases that have responded favorably to other treatment, therapeutic effect can be enhanced by selecting certain of these procedures. For example, for diseases of internal organs, exercise more on the head; for diseases of lower limbs, massage more on the back and legs.

1. Knocking the teeth
Close the lips lightly and knock the upper and lower teeth together rhythmically 30 to 40 times.
2. Cleaning the mouth
Close the lips lightly. Use the tongue to sweep the space between the teeth and lips. Start with the left side, then do the right, 30 times each.
3. Rubbing the hands
With the palms facing each other, rub them forcefully together from a slow to a fast pace, 30 to 40 times until heat is felt.
4. Touching the face
Use the warm palms resulting from rubbing to touch the face on the left, then move across the forehead and down to the right, 7 to 8 times. Repeat from the opposite direction another 7 to 8 times.

* Translated from *Acupressure Therapy,* An Fai Medical College, published by Commercial Press, Hong Kong, 1973.

5. Massaging the eyes

Use knuckles of the index, middle, and ring fingers to massage along the orbits (sockets) of the two eyes. First massage from the medial side to the lateral side, then from the lateral side to the medial side. Repeat each procedure 7 to 8 times.

6. Massaging the Tai-yang point (in the depression about one inch from the lateral corner of the eye)

Use the tips of the middle fingers to press and massage the Tai-yang points on both sides of the head in a rotary motion, first clockwise and then counterclockwise. Repeat in each direction 7 to 8 times.

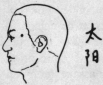

7. Wiping the forehead

Use the tips of the middle fingers to wipe laterally from the middle of the eyebrows, moving slowly to the hairline. Do it 7 to 8 times.

8. Pushing the head

Use Yu-chi (on the surface of the palm at the middle of the first metacarpal bone) to hold the sides of the head. Push from the anterior hair-edge to the posterior hair-edge (at the nape of the neck). Do it 30 to 40 times.

9. Pressing Pai-hui (five inches back from the middle of the middle front hairline), Feng-fu (one inch above the back hairline at the nape of the neck), and Ta-chui (see under Common cold)

Use the tips of two middle fingers to massage the above points one by one in the sequence given. Massage each point for about one minute.

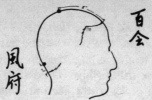

10. Vibrating the ears

Place the four fingers of each hand at the occipital region (back) of the head with the palms firmly over the auricular (ear) canal. Then rapidly and rhythmically vibrate the palms against both ears, 30 to 40 times.

11. Finger-knocking at the post-auricular region

Place the four fingers of each hand at the occipital region with palms pressing firmly over the ear canal. Then, use the index and middle fingers to knock at the occiput (back skull) bilaterally until one can hear the sound "Dong" distinctly. Repeat about 20 times.

12 Slapping the chest

With the fingers of both hands extended, use the fronts of the fingers to slap the chest (coordinate your inspiration with the slapping). Repeat 7 to 8 times.

13. Rubbing the flanks

Use the Yu-chi area of both hands to rub against the flanks bilaterally. The motion should be rapid. Repeat 30 to 40 times.

14. Massaging the abdomen

Place the left hand on the navel, then place the right hand upon the left hand. Push with force in a clockwise direction, 30 to 40 times.

15. Rubbing the back

Hold both hands as fists. Use the four meatcarpophalangeal joints (knuckles) of each hand to press against the back bilaterally. Rub upward and downward. Motion has to be rapid, with power, 30 to 40 times.

16. Hitting the spine and sacrum

Hold both hands as fists. Use the metacarpo-phalangeal joints to hit along the edges of the spine bilaterally. Raise fists as high as possible up the spine and move them down to the sacrum while hitting. Hit downward and upward 3 or 4 times.

17. Rubbing the thighs

Sit upright on a flat surface with legs crossed. Use both palms to rub against each thigh, 30 to 40 times respectively.

18. Clasping the calves

Sit with legs crossed on a flat surface. Use fingers to clasp the gastrocnemius (calf muscle) working from above down to the Achilles tendon. First do the left calf, then the right one.

19. Rubbing the Yung-chuan point (see under Fainting)

Use the edge of a palm to rub rapidly and powerfully against Yung-chuan, 30 to 40 times, until the center of the foot feels warm. Start with the left foot, then do the right one.

20. Respiration

Stand up with a shoulder-width distance between feet. Raise both hands (palms facing upward) from the abdomen to the larynx region. Simultaneously raise your head, stretch your back, and inhale. Then bring both hands (palms facing downward) from the larynx region back down to the abdomen region, and at the same time bend the head back and exhale. During exhalation, make the four sounds: "Ha, A, Hsi, Shi." Repeat two times.

ACUPRESSURE FOR MAINTAINING HEALTHY EYES *

The following exercises need to be done twice daily (once in the morning and once in the evening). Every procedure should be repeated 20 times. They can also be performed once after a prolonged period of using the eyes (for example, after continuous reading of books).

1. Massage of upper ocular orbits

Use the front surface of the left and right thumbs. Place them upon the upper orbits (sockets) of each eye beneath the eyebrows (at trigger points, or points where pain is experienced). The other four fingers of each hand form a bow along the forehead. Use two thumbs to massage gently over the trigger points. Do not use excessive force.

2. Pressure massage of nose root

Use the thumb and index fingers of either hand to press on the lateral ends (sides) of the nose root (i.e., on Ching-ming points). First massage downward, then press upward. Repeat the procedure.

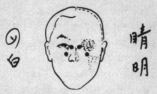

3. Massage of cheeks

Use the front surface of both left and right index fingers to press approximately at the center of the left and right cheeks (about the position of Szu-pai points). Use the left and right thumbs to support the mandible

* Translated from *Acupressure Therapy*, An Fai Medical College, published by Commercial Press, Hong Kong, 1973.

at its depressions. The other three fingers of each hand are held in the form of a fist. Use the index fingers to massage the central points of the cheeks continually.

4. Pressure massage around ocular orbits

The left and right index fingers are bent like bows. Use the medial surface of the second phalangeal joint (knuckle) of each finger, pressing it firmly against the upper orbit. Thumbs should press against the Tai-yang area (temples). The other fingers of each hand are held as a fist. During the procedure, press the second phalangeal joint (medial surface) against the orbit from above and move downward and up in a circular motion. At the same time, thumbs are massaging the Tai-yang points. Repeat the procedure.

About the Author

Pedro Chan is an acupuncture research associate at the White Memorial Medical Center, Los Angeles, and a visiting lecturer at the School of Acupuncture, Acupuncture Research Institute, Los Angeles, and Pacific Hospital, Long Beach. Currently, he is editor of the *Acupuncture News* bulletin. He comes from a traditional Chinese medical family; his father is a doctor in Macao. Chan is also the author of *Wonders of Chinese Acupuncture* and *Electro-acupuncture—Its Clinical Applications in Therapy*. He is a charter member of the Acupuncture Research Institute, Los Angeles, a member of the American Acupuncture and Herb Research Institute, Los Angeles, and a member of the Kowloon Herbalist Association in Hong Kong.